I0839661

Fitness Motivation

Top 20 Motivation Tips to Get in Shape

By
Bring on Fitness

© **Copyright 2018 – Bring On Fitness – All rights reserved.**

The contents of this book may not be reproduced, duplicated, or transmitted without direct written permission from the author.

Under no circumstances will any legal responsibility or blame be held against the publisher for any reparation, damages, or monetary loss due to the information herein, either directly or indirectly.

<u>Legal Notice:</u>

This book is copyright protected. This is only for personal use. You cannot amend, distribute, sell, use, quote, or paraphrase any part or the content of this book without the consent of the author.

<u>Disclaimer Notice:</u>

Please note the information contained in this document is for educational and entertainment purposes only. Every attempt has been made to provide accurate, up-to-date, complete, and reliable information. No warranties of any kind are expressed or implied. Readers acknowledge that the author is not engaging in the rendering of legal, financial, medical, or professional advice. The content of this book has been derived from various sources. Please consult a licensed professional before attempting any techniques outlined in this book.

By reading this document, the reader agrees that under no circumstances is the author responsible for any losses, direct or indirect, which are incurred as a result of the use of information contained within this document, including, but not limited to, errors, omissions, or inaccuracies.

About Bring On Fitness

Our passion for fitness gave life to **Bring On Fitness**. We started with the goal of helping as many people as we can. To educate, motivate and to help change peoples lives for the better. Bring On Fitness is not only for the fitness enthusiasts, but also for the beginner. We strongly believe nothing is more important than learning the basics and creating a strong foundation in both nutrition - through meal planning, and in exercise - by following a specific plan. This is just as important for the beginner, as it is for the experienced athlete.

We set high standards for ourselves, the information we share, and the products we carry. Our goal is to provide you with exceptional products that suit your needs and the knowledge and motivation to help you work towards and achieve your health and fitness goals.

Check us out at www.bringonfitness.com

“Our Mission is to have a positive impact in changing peoples lives. We will deliver the best possible fitness and nutrition solutions that will empower people to achieve their health and fitness goals.”

Table of Contents

Introduction

I would like to thank you for purchasing this book, "Fitness Motivation: Top 20 Motivation Tips to Get in Shape." The title may be a good indicator of what we are going to try to achieve through this book – motivating you to get into shape.

This book is about you and making you the fitter version of yourself that you always wanted to be. It might seem like you have tried several options and just haven't been able to achieve the degree of success you wanted to, but this book is going to try to change that for you.

Many people in the world are living the kind of lifestyle we've become accustomed to living, lamenting about the fact that they just don't know how to get fitter, even though they want to. It is a common health challenge that all of us face in the world today and is something that becomes even more important given the kind of lifestyle disorders we are growing used to seeing.

However, losing weight or getting in shape is not easy. While the task itself is a journey on its own, many of us also realize that we don't have ways to motivate ourselves to keep trying to achieve these goals constantly. As a result, many people tend to give up on fitness soon after giving it a shot.

I'm here to tell you that things can indeed be different. Through the course of this book, we are going to focus on several tips of interest, which you can implement in your life. The idea is that you will not only change the way you see fitness but also change the way you see yourself. Fitness isn't just about getting yourself in shape physically. It also happens to be an emotional labor of love.

Thus, this book focuses on both aspects of getting you into shape. After all, you cannot achieve one without the other, and we want the effect to be as well-rounded as possible.

So what are you waiting for? Let us get started on this journey toward better health and fitness. Happy reading!

Thanks again for purchasing this book. I hope you enjoy it and it brings you value!

Chapter One: Getting Started

Fitness Tip #1: Write Down What's Stopping You

By now, you have decided to commit toward being fit. Already, there might be a tiny part of your brain that is telling you this isn't the best idea for you and might be giving you several reasons why not. Your mind might try to convince you that you are too busy for this or that you have not been able to successfully stick to a workout routine in the past. In fact, your mind might tell you all sorts of things that might seem very convincing at first.

This is where writing it down helps you to put those words on a piece of paper. They now make a list of reasons why these things cannot possibly work for you. Now, look at the paper as though it were somebody else's list of reasons – would you be as easily convinced of the decision not to work out? Probably not. By writing this down, you will realize that you're stopping yourself from achieving something that is truly possible. This will help you focus on the important part, getting to set goals for yourself – minus the excuses – this time around.

Fitness Tip #2: Write Down Your Goals

It seems like in the beginning of this motivational journey, you have a fair bit of writing to do – and for a good reason. It not only serves as a way for you to view your reality more objectively, but it is also a physical reminder of things that you want to have. Think about it like you would while writing a shopping list. Doesn't remembering all the things you want to buy become so much easier when you have a list to help you with the process? You're no longer tempted to stray away from the list and buy things you don't necessarily need – and you avoid regret.

Writing down your goals will have a similar effect – it saves you from getting too distracted or from spiraling into the kind of changes you want to see with a level of immediacy. Instead, write down two goals – yes, just *two* to begin with. This is a realistic number to work toward and will make sure that you are not pulled into to too many directions. Thus, you will be able to keep your eyes on the prize at all times.

Fitness Tip #3: Write Down Why These Goals Matter

Speaking of keeping your eyes on the prize, you want to write down why this goal is important to you. There is a larger perspective that's always involved in goal setting, and you want to note that down and keep it somewhere you can see it. This way, on your bad days – or on those days when you don't feel particularly inspired – you have the option of looking at these reasons and reminding yourself exactly why you got into this in the first place.

Psychologically speaking, doing this is important. This is because the human brain is a creative and imaginative thing – and when it conspires to work against you, you might find that you can think of so many reasons not to stick to the workout you planned. This is not a good sign, and you want to be able to beat that. Hence, note those goals down. Maybe use them as a reminder when you wake up every morning to make sure they're etched in your memory – and in your habits.

Fitness Tip #4: Create Goals for the Week

As important as it is to keep your eyes on the prize at all times and to keep in mind the larger picture at play here, you also need to focus on the smaller things. Too much ruminating about the future of your goals and whether or not you will be able to achieve them can create a sense of dysphoria with your current self. Moreover, you will be putting in the hard work, so you will want to look at the kind of results that make sense to you.

Quite simply, this means you need to create two separate timelines for your goals - the goals you initially noted down are goals you want to achieve in the long term, perhaps over months of getting into shape. At the start of each week, on the other hand, you might want to set goals for yourself going into the week. This will mean you set a relatively small but achievable goal for that week. When you look back, you will have achieved it already, and this should remind you that you will be able to achieve your broader goals as well!

Fitness Tip #5: Chain Your Events and Goals

This tip works on two separate levels – that of your events on a particular day, as well as the larger goals that you have set. Link your weekly goals to your overall goal. The successive chaining of your weekly goals should lead up to the larger goal that you set for yourself, and the kind of goal we are talking about is left to your discretion. For instance, if you embark on a plank challenge and set your goal as 1 minute for a particular week, try to keep that in line with your monthly goal. Maybe you want to achieve a five-minute plank by the end of the month. This will happen in small increments that you will chain together to achieve the larger picture.

Similarly, another kind of chaining can occur in your daily life – that of your events. When you chain your events, it's like you are creating a pattern of habits for yourself. By doing so, you will ensure that you cannot postpone a scheduled workout by making excuses because you already have something else planned for later.

Fitness Tip #6: Follow Your Plan!

Now, you've gone through all of that work to make a plan that you can follow to achieve the goals that you want to. You've made sure that the goals align at different levels and that any means of excuse cannot postpone your workout. What's next? Well, to follow your plan, of course! This might seem like a silly thing to talk about. Why else would you make a plan if not to follow it? But implementation is the part that a lot of people tend to struggle with, and we need to make sure that you don't have the same problem.

Some people find it helpful to stick reminders of their workout plan throughout the house, using post-it notes. Others set reminders or alarms on their phones. There are different ways to make this consistency work for you. What matters at the end of the day is that you *are* being consistent and not backing out. This might come in the form of setting smaller, more realistic goals at the start and not getting too ambitious – or just through persevering through the odds. Whatever it may be, find what works for you, and make sure you stick to it – and follow your plan!

Chapter 2: Action Plans

Fitness Tip #7: Don't Skip Days

We've all had the odd lazy morning where we wake up and convince ourselves that we do not necessarily need to work out immediately. There is always the option of *later*. It is this "later" that tends to be the bane of several fitness enthusiasts, which happens because they give themselves too much room to create this option. You don't want to do that – convince yourself later isn't an option. If you skip one day, that one day can quickly turn into two, two into three, and you will run the risk of slipping back into your old lifestyle and habits.

This will mean that workouts will need to happen on days even when you don't feel particularly "in the mood" for them. You simply need to suck it up and do it – nine out of ten times, you will be feeling better at the end of a workout anyway. Of course, there are special circumstances, such as an illness or an injury, which you should be careful about, and on those days, make sure you don't push yourself. Otherwise, however, keep it up!

Fitness Tip #8: Create Exercise Intervals

Here's the thing – I get it. All of us are on a schedule; it can get difficult to find an hour-long slot during a day to set aside for a workout. This becomes a common reason that working professionals ending up not working out (pun intended), because they tend to think, "I simply don't have the time." If you are one of those people who have shied away from fitness regimes for this reason, I want to tell you that you are wrong.

It is possible to make time to fit in your regime, and this does not have to be a burden on the rest of your daily schedule.

The simple solution to this situation is creating exercise intervals. An hour in one slot doesn't seem possible? Make it two slots of half an hour each, or maybe three slots of 20 minutes each. Split these slots throughout the day, so you're able to complete them whenever a pocket of time opens up for you. That way, exercising won't feel like so much of a strain. Moreover, pockets of exercise throughout the day will make sure that you feel energized and motivated to tackle whatever comes next!

Fitness Tip #9: It's a Number Game

You will have noticed that your goal setting happens in the form of numbers. To put it simply, "By X time, I want to be able to do this Y times," or "By the end of the month, I want to lose X pounds." This quantifies your relationship with exercising and makes a fitness regime that much easier to monitor. You want to be able to monitor your progress, as you will know how close or far you are from achieving your goals – and make any necessary changes that will make the process easier for you.

To do this, also keep a record of your body stats. By this, I do not mean weight – our weight can fluctuate several times during a single day and thus is not viewed as the best marker that you are meeting your goal. Instead, take body measurements each week – at the same location and at the same time of the day – so that you know everything else is constant. Track your body fat percentage, if you feel like that might help. Track the number of calories you take in versus the number of calories you burn through your workout. All of this will give you a more holistic picture of whether or not you are meeting your goals.

Fitness Tip #10: Have a Fitness Buddy

Most things are much easier to do when you have company to help you through the process. This becomes particularly important when you are working out. While working out alone can feel like a chore, working out with somebody else can feel like a breeze and is often a lot of fun. Whatever activity you do choose to do, try to find someone else who is also interested in that activity to make that regime something to look forward to. The other person may also similarly benefit from having someone to share their workout with.

This will help keep you on track because you aren't just accountable to yourself anymore. You also need to keep in mind somebody else's schedule. This will make sure you aren't late for workouts or don't miss them. At the same time, you are ensured of a fun workout with someone who understands exactly what struggles you are going through with your fitness regime. You will be able to support and motivate each other constantly to achieve your respective goals!

Fitness Tip #11: Be Inspired, Don't Compare

We live in the times of social media, where content is constantly bombarded at us. There is no way to avoid it. It has taken over several parts of our lives and is perceived as integral. At the same time, you will notice that the choice to target content specific to some social media users has also been rising constantly. This means that each person is now forced to consume a particular kind of social media content, whether they like it or not. In this time, you will notice that your newfound liking for fitness regimes will also reflect in what is displayed to you on social media.

Invariably, you will try to compare your process and journey to that of others – because it does tend to feel like the others are always doing so much better. But that isn't true – they are probably looking at your journey and thinking the same about you. You need to remember not to compare your stories with each other, as each of you has a different history and a different challenge going on. Instead, be inspired by each other; look at the work they're putting into the task – look at what works and what doesn't. Learn from them!

Fitness Tip #12: Have Your Friends Help

Remember those goals that I told you to note down, so you are constantly reminded of what you want to achieve? Well, this tip works along similar lines as well. Instead of just writing it on a piece of paper, I want you to tell your friends what you are aiming to achieve and why. This process of sharing with your friends will make your journey easier as they are there to help you through it. Moreover, they will also be around to constantly remind you of the goals you set for yourself – even if you think you may forget.

Importantly, we all have our bad days when we feel like nothing seems to be going our way. On these days, it can be particularly difficult to believe in yourself and think that you can achieve the goals you set out to do. This is where your friends will come in. They are going to provide much-needed perspective and relief in your life by reminding you of how far you've come and by motivating you the rest of the way. And if they think you can do it, you better believe that you can do it!

Chapter 3: Other Sources of Support

Fitness Tip #13: Pro tips are pro-tips!

Whatever kind of fitness regime you are looking to follow, there are probably several people out there who do it as well. This is a good reminder that you are not alone on this journey. In addition to this, what you should try to do is find people in your area of interest who inspire you. Marathon runners, fitness bloggers, vloggers, and other such experts can have a lot to say about the process of becoming fit – and they know. They've not just gone through the process themselves, but they've seen countless others go through it as well.

They know what works, what doesn't, what can be a little difficult, what you will be able to ease past, common mistakes that others made, and so on, and so forth. As somebody starting your fitness journey, this can be very useful information. Moreover, you will soon find that your expert will be someone you not just *listen* to but also look up to and are inspired by. This *will* make a difference in your journey.

Fitness Tip #14: Have Tangible Proof of Your Progress

Alright, you already know that taking measurements and noting down the numbers is a good way to track your progress – it gives you a quantifiable means to understand it. While this tip is good in and of itself, we also don't possess the capacity to understand numbers in their absolute. Your body fat percentage may be down by 3%, but what does that mean to you? What is the solution to this? Take pictures.

Take pictures of your progress at regular intervals – at the same time of the day, of course. You might not understand the numbers yet, but the pictures will show you the difference between your past and current self. Having such tangible proof of the changes that you are going through can be quite helpful and inspiring. The changes that you see in yourself and all the little things that make you proud of that photo – and how far you've come – all matter! This will motivate you to push yourself further and to do better!

Fitness Tip #15: Find Other Victories

Sometimes, you will notice that despite putting in all the hard work, you don't seem to be losing weight. That weight goal that you set for yourself might look unattainable, but you know what? That's okay. A measure on a weighing scale is unlikely to tell you how far you've come. This is because of several reasons. First, given that your weight is likely to fluctuate throughout the day, it is not a reliable measure of your progress. Moreover, you might be losing weight in fat and still have the muscle mass to account for – and your scale doesn't know the difference!

This is why you need to find other victories for yourself. Think of all the other measures you take into consideration. Think about how much better your stamina has become, how little you crave unhealthy food now, and how your lifestyle has changed for the better. These are all your victories, too, and they deserve to be celebrated. Don't take that away from yourself!

Chapter 4: The Mental Game

Fitness Tip #16: Be More Mindful

As I said earlier, becoming fit is not just a matter of being in better physical health. You want to be mindful of your process as well. This is the only way that your mind and body will evolve in sync with each other. You don't just want to engage in the practice of exercise mindlessly and without giving any thought to it – you want to deeply engage with the process. This way, you're achieving a two-fold goal that takes into consideration not just your physical self, but also your spiritual self.

Understand how it changes your body and changes you. Notice the specific responses of your body to exercise; be more aware of what you are doing. Extend that awareness to the environment around you, and try to be inclusive of all these processes in your workout routine. You don't want it becoming a series of movements that you do just because you *need* to. This will help establish a more coherent connection with your actions and will stabilize them.

Fitness Tip #17: Words Can Be Inspiring

The pen is mightier than the sword, they say; this is very true even in the case of finding inspiration for your workouts. Think about it this way. Instead of punishing yourself for not exercising (the sword, in the analogy), what you want to do is focus on words that can help (ergo, the pen). There are several fitness bloggers, professional sportspeople, and trainers who have a lot to say about the rewarding journey of being fit.

Listen to what they have to say – you will find at least some of it inspiring.

Of the ones that particularly inspire you, choose a few to keep physical reminders of. Maybe these can work as a note on your fridge or on the nightstand where you place your glasses. Maybe you want to make a poster of it and put it up somewhere in your room. Do whatever works for you, and you will have a reminder of these inspiring words whenever you need them. Also, try to read a motivational quote daily, just to mix things up a little and add some novelty!

Fitness Tip #18: Imagine Your Success

To achieve success and to be more confident of your ability to achieve this success, think about your future self in your mind and *visualize* how this success in meeting your goal is going to change you. This technique has been used by experts and novices alike. The success of visualization has also been bolstered by numerous research studies that support it, indicating that this will give you the edge you need to help you perform and be *better*.

Imagine your success and think about your future self – now go ahead and give that future self an obstacle, and see how you respond to it. Keep practicing this so you can achieve the kind of success you envision.

However, like all good things, you need to remember to do this in moderation. You don't want to focus so much on the future that you lose sight of the present. Don't build castles in the air – this is why we focus on workable goals that you can achieve. Maintaining the balance between imagination and being grounded in reality will go a long way toward helping you achieve your goals.

Fitness Tip #19: Compete with the Past You

Competition can be motivating for a lot of people – there are the rewards and satisfaction of knowing that you did *better and* are *better* in a certain situation. Few things are more rewarding than achieving this with your past self – you want to be in constant competition with your older self. This is for two reasons. One, it ensures that you are not competing and comparing yourself with another person, which preserves the sanctity of your journey and keeps it your own, and two, you get to look back and see how far you've come, and it's a healthier kind of competition to engage in.

You can do this in one of two ways. First, all the tracking and recording and noting down of measurements will surely help you understand how far you've come. Additionally, with the technique of visualizing your success, you will also be able to make considerations for – or *imagine* - when you beat your past self and set a new personal record. The fun part of all this? Your past self will keep changing with time, so you don't run the risk of becoming stagnant or getting bored!

Fitness Tip #20: Be Patient

Yes, we all want to see results in our lives as quickly as possible, and it can get quite frustrating when the results don't show up when we want them to. This can be particularly difficult in the case of exercise – but you cannot allow it to demotivate you. You need to be patient with yourself and believe that you will see the results you want to see. However, all this will only happen with time. The process is not one with immediate results, and you already knew that. Mark off your little victories, they will soon begin to add up.

You will feel fitter soon enough, and that is something that can only happen if you give yourself the time to see those changes. Don't give up. You know you have it in you to achieve your goals. All you need is a little time, a lot of hard work, and a little bit of patience to top it all off. Good luck!

Conclusion

This concludes the much-needed motivational guide to fitness, designed to help inspire and motivate you through the process of becoming a healthier person. Thank you, yet again, for choosing this book for your journey – and I hope that it was as enriching and helpful as you needed it to be. Your successful fitness story will be a testament to the importance of this book.

It is not easy for anyone to get started on a new habit – and thus, I must laud you for trying. Things might initially seem like they are difficult, and you might just think that you need some extra guidance to keep you on track. This is where the book comes in – through giving you motivational tips that help you set your own goals and become aware of your progress. These tips give the agency and control of your life right back to you. Congratulations on regaining that control!

Through this book, by following the tips, and by staying motivated through it all, you will discover that you view yourself in a much more positive light. This is a victory you should strive to achieve at the same time as your physical fitness goals. As I mentioned earlier, these two goals go hand-in-hand. It is through this overall positivity and goal-oriented outlook that you are going to achieve the success you want. This won't just be limited to the area of fitness; it will soon apply to the rest of your life as well.

Thank you, and remember to share how well these motivation tips work for you. You can do that by writing a review in your Amazon account under Your Orders > Digital Orders.

26

Thank you,

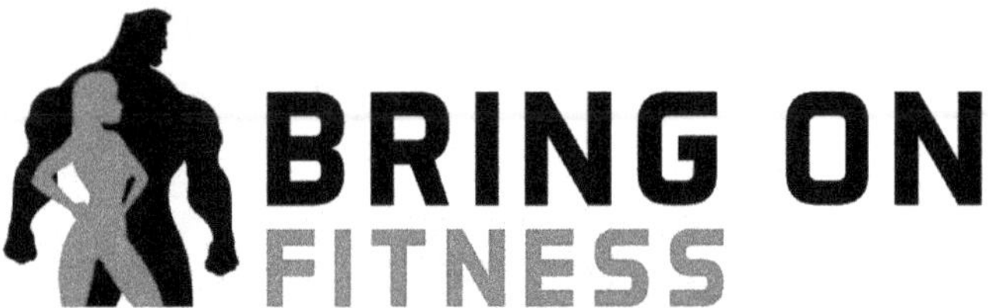

Sources

http://routineexcellence.com/fitness-motivation-tips/

https://www.webmd.com/fitness-exercise/features/fitness-top-10#1

https://www.fitnessmagazine.com/workout/tips/workout-motivation-tips/

https://www.realbuzz.com/articles-interests/fitness/article/top-10-motivational-tips-for-fitness/

www.ingramcontent.com/pod-product-compliance
Lightning Source LLC
Chambersburg PA
CBHW061926270726
48659CB00002BA/981